Bernhard Johannes Schmidt

Autism

and the
Refrigerator Mother Myth

A Rehabilitation of
Bruno Bettelheim

Contributions to the Psychology of
Science

Contributions to the
Psychology of Science

Bernhard J. Schmidt

Autism
and the Refrigerator Mother Myth

A Rehabilitation of Bruno Bettelheim

© 2019 Bernhard J. Schmidt,
Oberwarmensteinach
Alle rights reserved.

ISBN: 978-3749446469

Manufacture and Publisher:
BoD – Books on Demand, Norderstedt.

Bibliographic information from the German National Library:
The German National Library lists this publication in the
Deutschen Nationalbibliografie (German National Bibliography;
detailed bibliographic data can be found on the internet at
http://dnb.dnb.de.)

Inhaltsverzeichnis

I. Foreword...8

II. Historical context 10

   1 Treatment of autism 10

   2 Scientific positions 11

      2.1.a Rimland – Nature...13

      2.1.b Bettelheim – Nurture 13

    2.2 Vygotskij – KHK...14

   3 Therapeutic Positions..17

    3.1 Bettelheim "Successful therapy of autistic children"
....17

    3.2 Rimland: ABA...19

   4 Rimland and Lovaas..19

III. Problematic Perspectives of Bettelheim 23

   1 Concentration camp experience 23

   2 Stress and stimming...25

   3 Visceral stimuli / hyposensitivity 27

   4 Psychoanalytic perspective 29

   5 Abuse 31

IV. Correct Positions...35

V. The fight for interpretation sovereignty 36

   1 Bettelheim's criticism of Rimland 36

   2 Bettelheim's criticism of ABA 39

   3 Discrediting Bettelheim 40

3.1 Attack 1: the refrigerator mother myth 41

   3.1.a Evidence for the "refrigerator mother" 42

   3.1.b Evidence against 44

   3.1.c Summary 50

3.2 Attack 2: Doubts about the qualification / education of Bettelheim 50

3.3 Attack 3: Violent charges against Bettelheim 54

 4 Mixing science and parenthood 56

  4.1 Narcissism 57

 5 Distortion of the facts 60

VI. Look back..63

 1 Science turns into a dangerous myth 65

  1.1 Restriction of Therapeutic Approaches 67

  1.2 ABA as supposed "gold standard" 69

VII. Outlook..71

 Bibliography..72

Autism – and the refrigerator mother myth

I. FOREWORD

The "fridge mother" is one of the central myths in the field of autism research. And has always been associated with Bruno Bettelheim and his book "The Empty Fortress".

But that is a myth!

And it's a myth that has negatively impacted both autism research and the development of autistic support for more than 50 years.

According to my hypothesis, the discrediting of Bettelheim and his psychodynamic approach by the "fridge mother" myth have prevented any development. Just like the merry-go-round at the fair, so for 50 years the "research" rotate around the search for neuro-physiological causes.

And the "therapy" for autistic people has barely got beyond ABA (Applied Behavior Analysis).

Exceptions here are only the "child centered" approaches, which have developed in parallel to the "research" in some countries.

The following is a critical presentation of the approach of Bettelheim, without idealizing or glorifying it in any way. At Bettelheim there is a lot to criticize - but a "fridge mother" as a cause of autism is definitely not with him!

This is a myth that, according to another hypothesis, was set in the world by the adversaries of Bettelheim, especially Rimland and Lovaas.

I like to leave the review of this hypothesis to historians with appropriate training.

On the other hand, it is certain that the "fridge mother" myth has left the scientific level and shifted it to an emotional one.

Instead of scientifically checking Bettelheim's psycho-dynamic approach for his mistakes and strengths, it was from then on "Bettelheim insults the mothers / parents".

So if it says in the blurb of the edition of the 50th anniversary of Rimland's "Infantile Autism":

„He [Rimland] single-handedly realigned the field from a psychodynamic, parent-blaming perspective to a scientific, physiological course of action.“, then it is the exact opposite of the truth. With the myth of "parent-blaming", the scientific soil was definitely left. From today's point of view, it must be stated that Bettelheim was much closer to solving the autism puzzle than Rimland and Lovaas.

Highlighting the quotes always through me.

II. HISTORICAL CONTEXT

From today's point of view, many things seem strange, which was thought and made more than 50 years ago. Judging the thinking and actions of the people of that time with our present-day findings, this leads to a distortion of perception. The historical context, also to assess the performance of Bettelheim, is therefore to be considered.

1   Treatment of autism

In the 1960s, the "treatment" of children with mental disabilities or mental disorders took place in a very rudimentary and often cruel stage from today's perspective. This is how Bettelheim describes
„... *one, unbeknown to us when we accepted her, had been subjected to a long series of electroshock treatments a year before she came to us ...*" [Bettelheim (1967)]

An accommodation in "hospitals" where the "treatment" was often less squeamish and psychotherapeutic in any way was the rule rather than the exception. There were more or less „Verwahranstalten" [storage institutions].

9

„About a year later we learned that shortly after the withdrawal Laurie was committed to a state hospital for mentally defective children."
[Bettelheim (1967)]

The approach of the "Orthogenic School", which was headed by Bettelheim for many years, was really revolutionary for the time.

2   Scientific positions

Unlike in Russia, where Vygotsky developed a synthesis of nature and environment as early as 1929 [Vygotsky (1929)] through the "Culture Historical Concept", in Western Europe and the USA the nature and environment (nurture) were not only in the field Autism still thought of as largely exclusive opposites. Bettelheim is representative of the "Nurture" (environment), while his adversary Rimland is on the "Nature" side.

"Recently an ingenious analysis of all serious longitudinal studies available on human development was published by Bloom [1964]. It demonstrates in what ways, and how much, environment can influence certain human characteristics, particularly intelligence. It shows that the effects of an unfavorable environment act mainly

to arrest these characteristics, Some it may also deflect; but it cannot produce any traits that are not present in all human beings. "
[Bettelheim (1967)]

But Bettelheim does not exclude the discussion about hereditary, just does not consider these to be fruitful.

„*Even now, with the many research papers devoted to it, and with book-length reports such as Rimland's, Bosch's, and the present volume, **far too little is known about infantile autism to settle this question of organicity versus a psychogenic origin. As heuristic hypotheses both have value in the sense that by following both, no possibility is overlooked.** While I do not accept the hypothesis that autism is due to an original organic defect, I do not feel I can rule out its later appearance. On the contrary, I tend to believe that far from being organic in origin, infantile autism, when persisting too long, can have irreversible effects. This applies not to the affects - since we could restore full affective functioning to nearly all the autistic children we worked with for long enough – but to the intellectual or ego functions.*"
[Bettelheim (1967)]

2.1.a   Rimland – Nature

In 1964, three years before Bettelheim's book "The Empty Fortress," Rimland published the book "Infantile Autism: The Syndrome and Its Implications for a Neural Theory of Behavior." In this he develops a theory of autism as an inherited neurological defect. And rejects any psychodynamic approach. This position criticizes Bettelheim in "The Empty Fortress" very clearly (see also Chapter V. 1.).

2.1.b   Bettelheim – Nurture

Bettelheim does not rule out physiological causes, but argues that the understanding of inherited systems is less important for the understanding of human behavior.

„Unfortunately, because Kanner concluded that this disturbance is inborn, he failed to ask the question which, especially since Freud, we consider essential for understanding a psychological behavior; namely, Why does a person behave in this way instead of some other? Such a question cannot be avoided unless we assume that behavior is engaged in without the person's having any choice in the matter, as in the movements of a spastic.

12

But if one fails to ask this question, one fails to understand the person's motivation, and is easily tempted to ascribe to some inherent defect what does not make obvious sense in terms of conventional behavior."
[Bettelheim (1967)]

For Bettelheim, the investigation of all circumstances that can lead to the withdrawal of autistic children is in the foreground:

„What first disturbed me and aroused my interest in these children was how deliberately they seemed to turn their backs on humanity and society. If their experience of reality was such that it led to a total rejection, then there was a terribly important lesson to be learned about reality, or whatever part of it provoked their rejection. If we could understand which isolated aspects of reality were so abortive of humanity as to snuff it out, there might be something constructive we could do. "
[Bettelheim (1967)]

2.2   Vygotskij – KHK

It must be assumed that Vygotsky's "Cultural Historical Concept", which he had set out in 1929, inter alia in the "Fundamentals of Defectology", was unknown in Europe and the USA. Both through the World War and antagonistic political systems in West and East. For Vygotsky, who points out this mainly to blind and deaf-mute children, the central point was that an innate "defect" only becomes problematic in connection with the social environment with which enculturation occurs.

„If we subtract visual perception and all that relates to it from our psychology, the result of this subtraction will not be the psychology of a blind child. In the same way, the deaf child is not a normal child minus his hearing and speech. Pedology has long ago mastered the idea that if viewed from a qualitative perspective, the process of child development is, in the words of W. Stem, "a chain of metamorphoses" (1922). Defectology is currently developing a similar idea. A child in each stage of his development, in each of his phases, represents a qualitative uniqueness, i.e., a specific organic and psychological structure; in precisely the same way, a handicapped child represents a qualitatively different, unique type of development. Just as oxygen and hydrogen produce not a mixture of gases, but water, so too, says Guertler, the personality of a retarded child is something qualitatively different than simply the sum of under-developed functions and properties."
[Vygotskij (1929)]

14

How close Bettelheim and Vygotsky are in their positions, show quotes from the works of both:

„I use this example because it has also been observed how the mother of a blind or deaf child will let her infant grab the spoon and hold it with her; will enjoy his clumsy and ineffective efforts at helping her feed him and at feeding himself; will share his enjoyment of food though it gets messy around the mouth. In this way they establish mutuality around spoon-feeding although the blind child cannot see the pleasure on her face, nor the deaf child hear the pleasure in her voice.“
[Bettelheim (1967)]

„The unfortunate lot of the blind is not brought about by the physical condition of blindness, which by itself is not a tragedy. Blindness serves only as the ground for the onset of a series of tragedies. "Lamentations and sighs," Shcheihina ... describes an incident in a school for the blind when "the attendant had to feed an eight-year old boy with a spoon simply because his family never permitted him the opportunity of learning to eat by himself.“ [Vygotskij (1929)]

Had Vygotsky been known in the US, the dispute between Bettelheim and Rimland would almost certainly have been different.

3   Therapeutic Positions

On the basis of the very different positions between "nature" and "environment", of course, the therapeutic positions are divergent.

3.1   Bettelheim "Successful therapy of autistic children"

Bettelheim, based on a psychodynamic approach, relies on the creation of a favorable environment for the development of (mentally disturbed) children.
With this approach, he is far ahead of the time.

„Er will keine Heilung um jeden Preis, keine oberflächliche Symptombehandlung, kein gewaltsames Herausreißen des autistischen Kindes aus seiner verrückten Innenwelt. Seine Erfolge gründen darauf, daß er Bedingungen für diese Kinder schafft, die es den Kindern selbst ermöglichen, in freier Entscheidung aus ihrer Welt herauszukommen. Erst wenn der Therapeut seinem Hochmut entsagt, besser wissen zu wollen, wie

diese Kinder leben sollen, und seine Aufgabe darin sieht, den Kindern zu helfen, ihren Weg zu finden – erst dann, wenn sie diesen Weg gefunden haben, kann die Therapie zu einem Erfolg führen." [Stork, Jochen, Vorwort zu Bettelheim (1967)

"He does not want healing at any cost, no superficial treatment of symptoms, no violent ripping out of the autistic child from his crazy inner world. His successes are based on creating conditions for these children, which allow the children themselves to come out of their world in free choice. Only when the therapist renounces his arrogance to want to know better how these children are to live, and sees his task in helping the children to find their way - only when they have found this way, the therapy can become one Lead success."]

With his psychodynamic, environmental therapeutic approach, Bettelheim is a forerunner of the few child-centered support programs for autistic children today.

"In most institutions I know of the basic approach, even to the psychotic child, is to encourage him to see the world as it really is, which is exactly what the psychotic child cannot do. Instead, our task as we see it is to create for him a world that is totally different from the one he abandoned in despair, and moreover a world he can

enter right now, as he is. This means, above all, that he must feel we are with him in his private world and not that he is once more repeating the experience that "everyone wants me to come out of my world and enter his." How, then, is this done?"
[Bettelheim (1967)]

3.2   Rimland: ABA

Based on autism as an inherited neurological defect, Rimland is very close to the behavioristic approach of Lovaas (ABA - Applied Behavior Analysis).
„Bernard Rimland, a psychologist and parent of an autistic child, joined other parents to found the National Society for Autistic Children (now the Autism Society of America) [ASA] to promote intensive behavioral interventions that have evolved to become the goldstandard treatment for autism." [Baker (2010)]

4   Rimland and Lovaas

Rimland and Lovaas, together with parents of autistic children, founded the "Autism Society of America" (ASA) back in 1965, two years before Bettelheim's "The Empty Fortress." So not, as often misrepresented, only as a result of the book of Bettelheim!

*„The Autism Society of America (ASA) was founded in 1965 by Bernard **Rimland** and Ivar **Lovaas** together with Ruth C. Sullivan and a small group of other parents of children with autism. Its original name was the National Society for Autistic Children; the name was changed to emphasize that children with autism grow up. It is the oldest and one of the largest grassroots organization in the autism community with over 50,000 members and supporters connected through a network of nearly 200 chapters in the United States. The ASA's goal is to increase public awareness about autism and the day-to-day issues faced by people with autism as well as their families and the professionals with whom they interact. The organization advocates for programs and services for the autism community, and is a leading source of information, research, and reference on the condition."*
[Source: en.wikipedia.org]

19

Bettelheim, on the other hand, has criticized both the theoretical position of Rimland and the ABA approach Lovaas', both foundations of the ASA, in his book.

In the wake of the founding of the ASA and the postponement of the Nature / Nurture dispute on the emotional level of "parent-blaming", science loses its independence and ceases to be science.

„Parents of autistic children have lobbied Congress for research funding and formed major foundations of their own (such as Autism Speaks, founded by an executive and grandparent of an autistic child) to promote research. ***At a moment in time when the polarization over vaccines has created a deep rift between many parents and professionals, it is worth viewing today's conflict from the vantage point of history.*** *Forgotten for the most part by physicians, the memory of the refrigerator-mother explanation of autism has fundamentally shaped the autism community. It is a story that continues to stand as a warning to the danger of shutting out the voices of parents in the name of a persuasive theory."* [Baker (2010)]

Because something supposedly (!) went wrong in science, can parents make all the mistakes of this world without having to justify themselves in any way ?! They

20

are declared "experts".

This has led - and still does today - to the multitude of errors, e.g. the cause of autism concerns.

Rimland itself was e.g. one of the representatives of the "vaccinations as the cause of autism" theory, which holds up to this day by the "parent experts" against better knowledge.

It does not even surprise if all kinds of other cures, diets and remedies (such as MMS) can be propagated uncritically until today.

It is a reversed world where well-educated and critically endowed scientists are no longer the experts, but the parents.

Why do you still need educators, psychologists, doctors ... when parents are the better experts?

For what youth welfare offices, educational counseling centers ...?

As a result of the "fridge mother" myth, it was no longer critically researched what was right and helpful, but only what the parents like.

When Waterhouse (2013) writes

„Bishop (2010) reported that autism prevalence and severity are comparable to those of Down syndrome, yet funding autism is six times the amount allocated to study Down syndrome. Bishop also noted, 'the slope showing

increase of NIH funding over time is dramatically higher than for any other condition."

this is almost certainly due to the strong influence that parent associations such as the ASA and "Autism speaks" have on research.

And the researchers have joined without resistance, have willingly left the soil of science.

Have given up the independence, and complied with the dictates of alleged parents-experts.

III. PROBLEMATIC PERSPECTIVES OF BETTELHEIM

There are some things to criticize about the ideas and positions of Bettelheim, which I do not want to miss. Science does not mean to do everything right, but to face a critical discourse.

This was then refused Bettelheim. Now it is time to catch up.

1 Concentration camp experience

Bettelheim brings in his theoretical considerations very strong his concentration camp experiences. What is more than understandable on the one hand, on the other hand is also a hindrance. It often seems very constrained and as a projection of his experiences on the situation of autistic children.

„To know that one can interrupt an experiment at will keeps the ex|)crience from being totally overwhelming. It is precisely the irrevocable, more than the prospect of torture or death, that so destroys personality. The very fact that one submits to experiment in order to further a scientific inquiry can be enough. So much does it bolster

23

the self-respect that this alone can keep the experience from being shattering."
[Bettelheim (1967)]

He ignores the huge difference between children who first grow into the world and society through social interaction and adults who have been torn out of their already solidified world and put into a concentration camp.

„On the other hand, just as the "institutional" setting was the same for all the children Spitz studied [1945, 1949], though not all of them became vegetating children, so the conditions in the concentration camp ^ere more or less the same for all prisoners though not all men responded alike. One could observe in the camps virtually all types of schizophrenic adaptations and symptomatology – so much so that a description of prisoner behavior would amount to a catalogue of schizophrenic reactions."
[Bettelheim (1967)]

The parallels then appear very artificial:

„The moslem who let the SS get hold of him, not just physically but emotionally too, went on to internalize the SS attitude that he was less than a man, that he was not

24

to act on his own, that he had no personal will. But having transformed his inner experience to accord with his outer reality he ended up, though for entirely different reasons, with a view of him.scif and the world very similar to that of the autistic child." [Bettelheim (1967)]

2   Stress and stimming

Bettelheim also did not recognize the significance of stress in autistics. As shown in Schmidt (2015), stress is one of the main problems in autistic people besides anxiety.

„According to Selye's [1956] theory of the stress syndrome, for example, they should suffer from total exhaustion because their stress is unending. But this they do not. On the contrary, their defenses are powerfully backed up by energy. None of this energy is spent on assimilating or adapting to reality as we see it. In our terms they do little or nothing at all. Instead, all energy is funneled into the single defense: to blot out all stimuli, inner and outer, in order to avoid further pain or the impulse to act." [Bettelheim (1967)]

The "defensive measures" thus serve to reduce both stress and anxiety. It creates an overviewable and understandable world.

„*Inactive as she was Marcia had nevertheless, and long before she came to us, developed a twiddling behavior, a rapid shaking of one or two of her fingers. Often the twiddling was self-hypnotic. So was her staring at shiny, light-reflecting objects (such as a metal box) or most often at the ceiling with its light fixtures. Looking up at the ceiling she seemed to have particularly frightening hallucinations. Occasionally she put her hand flat to her face or nose. Perhaps she did this to make sure where her body ended, since in hallucinating she may have felt it extended to the images she projected on the ceiling. Or perhaps she did it to form a protective screen between her and a world she only dimly perceived, or what she hallucinated as being out there. Much later when she hallucinated this way she said, "See mom," and pleaded desperately, "Take mom away."*
Marcia's twiddling was not only self-hypnotic but also a discharge behavior, as if it were a compromise between the most primitive reactions of the animal or human being when confronted with imminent danger: to freeze or take flight. If anxiety mounts and neither device seems successful then a compromise ensues, a frantic and

aimless running back and forth. Marcia's body, frozen in total immobility, seemed to represent the first fright reaction. But the extremely rapid, back-andforth shaking of her fingers might be likened to the desperate, purposeless, back-and-forth running of the cornered animal who cannot or dares not take flight.“
[Bettelheim (1967)]

The psychoanalytic view of Bettelheim stands here, as usual, in the way of knowledge.

3   Visceral stimuli / hyposensitivity

Despite the description of various examples in which the children have a pronounced hyposensitivity in the area of visceral perception, Bettelheim fails to establish a connection.

„For example, a formerly mute autistic child who had recently acquired speech to the degree that she could fully understand, clearly respond, and express in complete sentences all she wished to say showed no pain reactions though she was obviously quite sick (high temperature, high white-blood count, etc.). Because, for a very short while, she had pulled up her leg in a way typical of children suffering from pain in the peritoneal

cavity, we suspected appendicitis. So the persons she felt closest to questioned her about pain in this region, and she was also examined for this daily by staff physicians of the University's department of pediatrics, including professors. But she showed no tenderness to palpation when examined, nor any rebound tenderness. ...
Mainly because she still showed no pain reactions whatever, nor did she protect the area, the medical decision was that it was not appendicitis."
[Bettelheim (1967)]

Thus, Bettelheim, along with his psychoanalytic perspective, comes to wrong conclusions.

„Quite a few autistic children, having reached this point, choose a particular way to further convince themselves it is really they who defecate. It seems that straining their muscles to push out the feces is not enough of a kinesthetic sensation to convince them that defecation happens only by their decision. So they add a deliberate doing: they dig the feces out of the rectum with their fingers. Our assurance that their bodies are well able to eliminate without manual help falls on deaf ears; they simply do not believe us." [Bettelheim (1967)]

The lack of sufficient visceral perception due to hyposensitivity is simply replaced by the sensation of the finger. No more and no less.

4   Psychoanalytic perspective

In particular, Bettelheim's psychoanalytic position, with its widespread speculation about alleged causes of children's behavior, is often misleading - and often hard to bear.

„From other autistic children we might have added many similar examples. I selected that of the ruptured appendix because it illustrates lack of normal reaction to visceral pain and because Mahler [1952] speaks of the "grossly inadequate peripheral-pain-sensitivity in these children" adding that "in contrast, proprioceptive stimuli, visceral pain, Was keenly felt and reacted to." But my example (and there were others) suggests that the lack of normal cathexis is not restricted to the periphery. I believe the difference is due to the difference in autistic withdrawal. Mahler's patient was only three and a half years old, while autistic mutism in a twelve-year-old (the age of our patient) reflects much more far reaching alienation than in a much younger child."
[Bettelheim (1967)]

If a hyposensitivity of the interoception, as also described by Bettelheim, is present, then this is largely sufficient as an explanation.

„This is further borne out by a type of behavior we have found in many—though not all—of our autistic children, namely their response to dentistry. And this, although we use only a dentist highly skilled and successful in treating even our most severely disturbed children.
Most of our autistic children have fought with inordinate strength, and with the violence of utter desperation even the gentlest of efforts to repair their teeth. Several of them showed no signs of discomfort though their teeth were rotting away, the nerves exposed. Though when questioned about it they gave no, or only the vaguest responses, and though they also understood that the dentist was there to relieve their pain, they so viciously fought off any intrusions in the mouth that they could not be treated. But I believe that had the children felt the pain enough :hey would have fought the dentist less, despite the meaning to them of the oral intrusion."
[Bettelheim (1967)]

Add to this the hypersensitivity of autistic people in the area of touch, hearing and smell, then the denial of treatment by a dentist, which is generally not experienced

30

as pleasurable, is understandable even without psycho-analytic speculation.

5   Abuse

Really worthy of criticism and at the same time catastrophic in the consequences is the overlooking of the abuse of children.

„*When she was about two and a half, constipation was so bad that from then on weekly enemas were forced on her, with the exception of a few intermittent periods when daily laxatives were used. The enemas she fought violently, and **as she grew stronger the father had to hold her down. This he did by lying down on the bed with her, face to face, holding her fast against his body while the mother-nurse administered the enema.** It was Marcia's first intimate bodily contact with a father who had otherwise hardly ever held the child or played with her, all of which highly eroticized the procedure. Much as she dreaded the enemas, they excited her. This, we believe, came to symbolize her central conflict. It made it ever more impossible for her to move at all and forced her even further into autistic withdrawal. The event she dreaded most—because her own body was made to violate her desire to hold on and was made to* *give out-was also what produced greatest sexual excitement. Moreover, the persons who thus excited her were seen as mortal enemies, while she was wholly dependent on them."* [Bettelheim (1967)]

Shifting the problems resulting from the abuse to the side of the victim (the child) by means of psychoanalytic speculation, instead of clearly identifying and preventing the abuse, is incomprehensible and unbearable from today's point of view.

„I might mention here that Pavenstedt [1956] reports on a boy whose speech temporarily "dropped out completely" at twenty-one months when for a few weeks he "was put through a ritual every evening be fore supper: the father at first held him down with his legs over his head while the mother gave him enemas or suppositories." Though the procedure was dropped after a few weeks, it was not until several months later, and after he had been encouraged to be more independent in other areas too that he "recommenced speaking, however his words were at last much less distinct than they had been [but] his withholding of feces for three or four days at a time . . . has persisted till now" that is, up to the age of twelve." [Bettelheim (1967)]

The physical and / or sexual abuse and its consequences are completely overlooked.

This completely misinterprets the child's actions.

„She sat on her bed for hours in a strange yoga position, her feet crossed under her, either motionless or excitedly rocking up and down. In this sitting position her rectum was certainly protected from intrusion; but in the rocking up and down she may have been trying to recreate the exciting anal stimulation of the enemas. At such times she was certainly concentrating on some inner sensations. Outwardly there was a strong, rhythmic change from quiet to highly aspirated breathing." [Bettelheim (1967)]

And yes, that can and must be criticized very clearly!

„When Joey came to us, going to the toilet like every other move in his life was surrounded by elaborate preventions. We had to go with him to the toilet; he had to take off all his clothes; he could not sit but only squat over the seat, and he had to touch the wall with one hand in which he clutched the tubes that powered his elimination. With his other hand he had to hold on to his penis when defecating, and close his anus when urinating. This was our first indication of how he feared that by opening his body too much he would lose all body

content, that all his "stuffing" would spill out. The terror he experienced when something left his body showed how fearful he was of losing anything from this closed system." [Bettelheim (1967)]

The description of protecting the penis and anus suggests much more of a previous abuse than of Bettelheim's psychoanalytic speculation. However, the historical context has to be considered.

IV. CORRECT POSITIONS

Despite all legitimate criticism of Bettelheim, which of course there are as well, a number of findings and positions of him are groundbreaking, or could have been. First, the psychodynamic approach to understanding autism.

From this derives the milieu therapy, which tries to create an environment in which the child can develop. And that on a long-term basis.

His early and sharp criticism of ABA can also be mentioned here.

But with the myth of the "refrigerator mother" and the subsequent massive impact of autism research by parent associations such as ASA and "Autism Speaks", these positive points and approaches were simply ignored.

V. THE FIGHT FOR INTERPRETATION SOVEREIGNTY

Bettelheim wishes, and this becomes very clear in his book "The Empty Fortress", a scientific discourse. But this is denied and instead a one-sided and bitter struggle for supremacy by all means begun.

Probably the extensive criticism of Bettelheim contributed both to Rimland's position and to ABA.

1   Bettelheim's criticism of Rimland

„Thus my essential disagreement with Rimland, for example, is not with his approach, but with his insistence that the psychogenic approach should be discarded; and this though he does not claim certainty for his ideas. I think it most important to investigate the hypothesis of an organic etiology. I can only wonder why he decries what he calls "the all too common practice of blatantly assuming that psychogenic etiology can exist or does exist" and that to do so "is not only unwarranted but actively pernicious."„ [Bettelheim (1967)]

Bettelheim, apparently after the appearance of "Infantile Autism" attached as an appendix to his book which is

certainly already in the process of being published,
tackles Rimland's position objectively.

*"A neurological theory of autism has indeed been
proposed by Rimland in a recently published monograph.
Since it is also, to my knowledge, the only book-length
report in EngHsh on infantile autism and the most recent
one at this writing—a German monograph will be
discussed later—I shall be referring to it again in this
chapter.*
**Rimland holds that the source of the autistic
disturbance is to be found in the reticular formation of
the brain stem. But a careful study of the evidence
presented in his book failed to convince me that autism
has anything to do with an inborn dysfunction of this or
any other part of the brain.** *And even if a specific
neurological dysfunction should some day be found to
correlate highly with the syndrome of infantile autism, it
would still be compatible with the psychogenic
hypothesis.*
*First, the possibility exists that if certain neural systems
are not appropriately stimulated within a specific period
of life, they may suffer permanent impairment. Hence the
absence of certain emotional experiences at a very early
age may account for the later dysfunction of some part of
the central nervous system.*

37

Second, and more important, we were able, through psychotherapeutic treatment, to reverse the course of the disturbance. As illustrated in this book by Joey's history, we have helped him and others to free themselves of all those symptoms that are viewed as typical of the disease, suggesting that infantile autism is not caused by an inborn dysfunction of the central nervous system. "
[Bettelheim (1967)]

„*I believe it is only because Rimland did not study autistic children carefully with the intention of deciphering the messages of their autism that he maintains they can do no more with their language than repeat what they hear others say.* ***He does not even discuss the fact that Kanner [1946], far from viewing the language of autistic children as a sign of inborn impairment, recognized it as meaningful to anyone who acquaints himself with the child's experience of reality.*** "
[Bettelheim (1967)]

Although this was subsequently attempted to deny, Bettelheim, as head of the "Orthogenic School", had very extensive and long-standing experience in dealing with not only autistic children at the time.

2   Bettelheim's criticism of ABA

Bettelheim also took a stand against ABA (Applied Behavior Analysis):

„Here I wish also to comment on current eflforts to deal with infantile autism through operant conditioning—that is, by creating conditioned responses through punishment and reward. Temporarily this breaks down the child's defenses against experiencing the frustrations of reality and arouses him to some action. But the actions are not of his devising. They are those the experimenter wants; that is, they are conditioned response actions. **Which means that autistic children are reduced to the level of Pavlovian dogs.**„
[Bettelheim (1967)]

The setting of the autistic child on the same level with animals, which criticized Bettelheim, we can still find today, for example, Tomasello (2006) [detailed review in: Schmidt (2015)].

„According to a recent description of operant conditioning [Lovaas, Berberich, Perloff, Schaeffer, 1966]:

39

Training was conducted six days a week, seven hours a day, with a fifteen-minute rest period accompanying each hour of training. During the training sessions the child and the adult sat facing each other, their heads about thirty cm apart. The adult physically prevented the child from leaving the training situation by holding the child's legs between his own legs. Rewards, in the form of single spoonsful of the child's meal, were delivered immediately after correct responses. Punishment (spanking, shouting by the adult) was delivered for inattentive, self-destructive, and tantrumous behavior which interfered with the training, and most of these behaviors were thereby supressed within one week." [Bettelheim (1967)]

And comes to the same result as Vygotsky:

„Speech in the sense of communication simply cannot be forced out of children. It can only be acquired as the outcome of personal relations. Forcing them into echolalia by bribing, shouting, or spanking will only lead to a greater dehumanization." [Bettelheim (1967)]

3   Discrediting Bettelheim

Instead of conducting a scientific discourse and developing a synthesis of the conflicting theories, such as in Vygotskijs KHK, the discrediting of Bruno Bettelheim was pursued. And this on three tracks.

3.1   Attack 1: the refrigerator mother myth

It is the "fridge mother" myth set in the world.

„Evans and Evans in their Dictionary of Contemporary American Usage [1957], and elaborating on Benedict's definition, state that "In sociology and anthropology, a myth is a collective belief that is built up in response to the wishes of the group instead of a rational analy.sis of the situation to which it pertains.""
[Bettelheim (1967)]

Through this, the scientific level of a critical dispute was abandoned and rushed against Bettelheim's alleged "blaming the parents".
But Bettelheim's descriptions were scientific case reports, factual statements of fact, not allegations or moral judgments.
Nevertheless, it is worth the effort to see if any clues can be found in the approximately 500-page book "The Empty Fortress" for a "refrigerator mother". And which passages rather speak against such a position of Bettelheim.

3.1.a   Evidence for the "refrigerator mother"

Without claim to completeness, here are some quotes that could indicate a "fridge mother" theory:

„Later, when writing with Eisenberg, his frequent collaborator, he [Kanner] went further in implying a relation between these children and their parents. In the same symposium [1955] in which I suggested that childhood schizophrenia might be a reaction to extreme situations, they [Eisenberg and Kanner, 1956] spoke of how "emotional refrigeration has been the common lot of autistic children." More explicitly, they said:

It is difficult to escape the conclusion that this emotional configuration in the home plays a dynamic role in the genesis of autism. But it seems to us equally clear that this factor, while important in the development of the syndrome, is not sufficient in itself to result in its appearance. There appears to be some way in which the children are different from the beginning of their extra-uterine existence. Indeed, it has been postulated that the aberrant behavior of the children is chiefly responsible for the personality difficulties of their parents who are pictured as reacting to the undoubtedly trying situation of having an unresponsive child. While we would agree that this is an important consideration, it cannot explain the social and psychological characteristics of the parents which have a history long anteceding the child.

It is difficult to see how the "emotional configuration in the home" can play "a dynamic role in the genesis of autism" if the child does not respond to it because he does not relate to people. The only way these two statements can be reconciled is to assume that the parents' behavior does not permit or induce the child to come out of his shell. That is, the only way one can accept Kanner's thesis that the home aflfects the disturbance and still hold his view that the child cannot relate would be to assume that the parents fail to evoke any response in the child and that he therefore remains in his original autistic state." [Bettelheim (1967)]

„*The mothers of autistic children are often described as cold and rigid, if not also intellectual. Certainly they are not free-moving in the realms of emotion or at least not in relation to their autistic child. In their emotions, then, many of them are nearly as frozen, nearly as rigid when they deal with the child as was Harlow's terrycloth mother.*" [Bettelheim (1967)]

43

With 500 pages you will certainly be able to find even more text passages, but none that would justify a more "fridge mother" myth and the publications based on it.

3.1.b   Evidence against

The passages that speak against the accusation, however, are diverse and show a very differentiated view of Bettelheim:

„Having said all this, it should be stated emphatically that no mother can, even at the start of her baby's life, adapt entirely to his needs, nor later adapt perfectly as he adjusts to her and the world. There will always be times when even the best and most responsive of mothers will expect too much of her infant, and at other times, or in other respects, too little. In the end she is a human being, variable and fallible. Were she not, her child would have little chance to test his adaptive capacities against reality, nor would her behavior ever challenge these to develop." [Bettelheim (1967)]

„Much as I have cautioned against the myth of the blissful infant, so I would caution here against the correlate myth of the perfect, all-giving mother we all wish we had had. Saints may be needed in heaven, but

44

they rarely make good parents. At least we hear little of their having had children or having raised them successfully."
[Bettelheim (1967)]

*"Here, as everywhere in life, fate plays a great and at times decisive role. **Infants are born with differing endowments, intelligence, temperaments. However great the influence of our earliest experience, and all later ones that build on them, they can only modify the endowment we are born with.** Inheritance is fate in this respect. A very fast mother will find it difficult to gear her rhythm to her very slow child even if she tries, because to move that slowly demands too large an adaptation of her."* [Bettelheim (1967)]

"In the meantime we had arranged for our two psychiatrists, who had followed Laurie's progress, to consult with the parents. Neither parent wished to talk with them, but finally agreed to, out of respect, as they put it, for the good work we had done with their child. Though they .said again that they recognized Laurie's progress, both parents listened impassively, the father without interest, to what we (the psychiatrists and I) had to say.

One of our psychiatrists summed up her impression of the interview by saying that throughout our talk with the parents, she felt they were so unwilling to listen to what we said that they probably did not hear us. We offered to keep Laurie at a fee agreeable to the parents but this was of no interest to them. I suggested they might call in a psychiatrist of their own choosing for further consultation. This did not interest them either. Whatever we said seemed to bore them. My belief is that this went deeper than mere disinterest. **Both parents had reached the end of their rope with Laurie. For years she had caused them to feel totally defeated as parents and by now they could afford to feel no more. Least could they afford to hope once more since they were convinced that to hope meant only to be the deeper disappointed later on.**

In reply to all arguments the father insisted that Laurie was his daughter and "the burden" he had to carry; the mother, that Laurie belonged to her and that therefore they had decided she would have to leave the School. When I reminded them of our agreement—that if we accepted Laurie she would be allowed to stay with us for as long as we felt was required—the father said, "I agreed because I was convinced you wouldn't keep her and that she's hopeless. Since she's made such progress . . ." and there he stopped." [Bettelheim (1967)]

The behavior of the parents could also have been interpreted much more unfriendly, e.g. as an expression of a narcissistic personality disorder.

„*My own belief, as presented throughout this book, is that autism has essentially to do with* **everything** *that happens from birth on; nor can we rule out the possibility that some prenatal deviation in development may be a contributing factor. But since I also believe that autism is basically a disturbance of the ability to reach out to the world, it will tend to become most apparent during the second year of life when more complicated contact with the world would normally take place.*"
[Bettelheim (1967)]

„*Because what we need to know is exactly how it comes about, in the lives of some children, that these vitally needed experiences do not occur. The controversy of what came first, the chicken or the egg (the child's or the mother's inability to respond to each other) seems fruitless. But neither is it answered by saying that the whole thing is the result of an interaction, which it certainly is.*
What we need to know are the minutiae of the steps in these interactions: what particular response to what particular event will, for example, result in autism

47

instead of neurosis; what are the specific intrinsic determinants in the infant that will predispose to autism instead of another type of childhood schizophrenia—or to no disease at all? Since all personality development, normal or abnormal, results from the interactions of a particular inheritance with a particular environment, to state that the interaction causes autism is a truism— unless, of course one subscribes to a simple hypothesis that autism is due only or mainly to an organic impairment **sui generis.** *It does not answer the question: What is the particular inheritance, and the specific environmental factor which, in their interaction, create autism?"* [Bettelheim (1967)]

„*There are some points on which I can agree with Rimland: one is that it serves no good purpose to make the parents of autistic children feel guilty as having caused the disturbance.* *Firstly, we cannot be sure that their attitudes and the handling of their infant was, in and of itself, sufficient cause. While we believe it to be a precipitating factor, this makes it only a necessary but not a sufficient condition. We cannot even be sure whether, or to what degree, they handled the child as they did because of his unusual responses to them. But even if it turned out one day that the parents' contribution is indeed crucial, they did as they did because they could*

48

not help themselves to do otherwise. They suffer more than enough in having such a child. To make them guilty will only add to the misery of all and help no one. **Nevertheless, it is one thing not to wish to make parents feel guilty because it makes them miserable and gains nothing for the child. It is another thing not to wish to find out what experiences may have caused or contributed to infantile autism, because to do so is "pernicious;" that is, may turn out to be painful to parents.**" [Bettelheim (1967)]

„Though never explicitly stated, childhood schizophrenia has been viewed as not much more than a negligible appendage of maternal pathology— occasionally so much so that reconstructions and study of the assumed cause of the disturbance (the mother) seem to have taken the place of the study of the disease itself. *And this is even more so in regard to the severest form of childhood psychoses, infantile autism. Direct connections have been established between maternal attitudes —about which relatively much was known, and which were easy to study—and the behavior of the schizophrenic child, about which little was known and which was difficult to understand.*" [Bettelheim (1967)]

49

3.1.c   Summary

Bettelheim was interested in a scientific discourse and answering questions about the genesis of autism. The depictions of Bettelheim on about 500 pages "Empty Fortress" are so differentiated that they can under no circumstances be subsumed under a simple "fridge mother".

Thus, the "refrigerator mother" is a false simplification in combination with a shift from the material to an emotional level "Blaming the mothers / parents". With the establishment of the "fridge mother" myth contrary to the facts, on the one hand, the scientific level of unbiased consideration was abandoned, and apart from Bettelheim also a psychodynamic approach was discredited.

3.2   Attack 2: Doubts about the qualification / education of Bettelheim

In addition to the "fridge mother" myth, doubts were voiced on the qualifications of Bettelheim. Again, the scientific framework is abandoned and the person is attacked.

„Although significant questions have been raised regarding Bettelheim's own credentials as a psychoanalyst,he did function as a public intellectual representing his profession in popular media. His story provides a bitter reminder that experts do not always listen and cannot always be trusted." [Baker (2010)]

As was the case with the "fridge mother" myth, here too the facts were ignored or reinterpreted in order to put Bettelheim in the worst possible light. Because:

„In den USA wurde Bettelheim zunächst Forschungsassistent an der University of Chicago. 1944 wurde er Leiter der dortigen „Orthogenic School" und Assistenzprofessor für Kinder- und Jugendpsychologie, -psychiatrie und -pädagogik. Die Einrichtung war von ihm so genannt worden, um die Kinder für ihren späteren Werdegang weniger zu stigmatisieren. Zu einem seiner dortigen Schwerpunkte zählte die Behandlung autistischer Kinder, wobei er eine eigene, psychoanalytisch geprägte Theorie über Ursache und Genese des Autismus entwickelte. An der „Orthogenic School" erarbeitete er mit der Unterstützung des Dekans der Chicagoer Universität, Ralph W. Tyler, die Milieutherapie, die wesentliche Weiterentwicklungen zu der bis

51

*dahin praktizierten analytischen Psychotherapie
hervorbrachte.*
*Ab 1952 bis zu seiner Emeritierung 1973 war er
ordentlicher Professor. 1971 wurde er in die American
Academy of Arts and Sciences gewählt."*
[Quelle: de.wikipedia.org
*Bettelheim initially became a research assistant at the
University of Chicago. In 1944 he became head of the
local "Orthogenic School" and assistant professor of
child and adolescent psychology, psychiatry and
education. The facility had been so named by him to
stigmatize the children less for their later career. One of
his focal points was the treatment of autistic children,
where he developed his own, psycho-analytically based
theory on the cause and genesis of autism. At the
Orthogenic School, with the support of the Dean of the
University of Chicago, Ralph W. Tyler, he developed the
milieu therapy, which produced significant advancements
to the previously practiced analytical psychotherapy.
From 1952 until his retirement in 1973 he was a full
professor. In 1971 he was elected to the American
Academy of Arts and Sciences.*]

The entry about Bettelheim in the English Wikipedia
reads as follows:

„After his death in 1990, it was discovered that he had substantially misrepresented his background and credentials. For example, he had never been a candidate at the Vienna Psychoanalytic Society and had only taken three introductory courses in psychology. His one PhD was in either aesthetics or art history (sources disagree). Bettelheim's theories on autism, for which he blamed parents and primarily mothers in The Empty Fortress (1967), raised controversy in his lifetime and are now considered to be discredited.

After his death, it was further revealed that Bettelheim often used violence against students who lived at the school even though he wrote against corporal punishment. Counselors at the school tended to merely perceive corporal punishment, whereas some but not all students perceived rage and out-of-control violence. Chicago-area psychiatrists were later criticized for knowing at least some of what was occurring and not taking effective action. The University of Chicago was also criticized for not providing their normal oversight during Bettelheim's tenure."
[Source: en.wikipedia.org/wiki/Bruno_Bettelheim]

It also has to be mentioned that the book "The Empty Fortress" was published by Bettelheim alone. But he did not work alone in the Orthogenic School, but was its leader. So there was a big team of doctors, psychologists ... at the side of Bettelheim. But to discredit Bettelheim, this had to be ignored.

3.3   Attack 3: Violent charges against Bettelheim

The efforts to discredit Bettelheim were thus beyond his death.

„Kurz nach Bettelheims Tod wurde Kritik laut, unter anderem erschien im amerikanischen Nachrichtenmagazin Newsweek ein Artikel mit dem Titel Benno Brutalheim. Bettelheim habe die Ergebnisse seiner wissenschaftlichen Arbeit gefälscht und Kinder in der Orthogenic School geschlagen, darunter auch Kinder mit Autismus.

Die „Züchtigungen" seien zum Teil spontan, öffentlich und aus für die Kinder nicht einsehbaren Gründen erfolgt, so die Aussage von ehemaligen Patienten. Etwa habe der Psychoanalytiker Bettelheim unbeabsichtigten Körperkontakt eines Kindes mit anderen Kindern beim gemeinsamen Sport als Manifestation unbewusster Aggression wahrgenommen. In Chicagoer Psychoanalytikerkreisen sei von Bettelheim daher schon

*Jahre vor seinem Tod als „Benno Brutalheim"
gesprochen worden.*

*Zu den Hauptkritikern zählt Richard Pollak, ehemaliger
Herausgeber des Magazins The Nation, dessen Bruder in
Bettelheims Obhut Suizid verübte. Zurückgewiesen durch
Bettelheim und mit den Hintergründen über den Tod
seines Bruders konfrontiert, stellt er in seiner Biografie
Bettelheims dessen Lauterkeit in Frage."*
[Quelle: de.wikipedia.org
*Shortly after Bettelheim's death, criticism became loud,
among other things appeared in the American news
magazine Newsweek an article entitled Benno
Brutalheim. Bettelheim had falsified the results of his
scientific work and beaten children in the Orthogenic
School, including children with autism.*

*The "chastisements" were partly spontaneous, public and
for reasons not visible to the children, according to the
testimony of former patients. For example, the
psychoanalyst Bettelheim perceived unintentional bodily
contact of a child with other children during sports as a
manifestation of unconscious aggression. In Chicago
psychoanalyst circles, Bettelheim had been spoken as
"Benno Brutalheim" years before his death.*

Among the main critics is Richard Pollak, former editor of the magazine The Nation, whose brother committed suicide in Bettelheim's care. Rejected by Bettelheim and confronted with the background of his brother's death, in his biography of Bettelheim he questions his sincerity.]

Without wanting to discuss the moral side of these attacks posthumously, let's just point out that a theory has to be examined independently of its spokesman - at least in science.

Even if Bettelheim had been the worst person in the world, that would not mean that his theory is wrong.

A detailed text on the allegations against Bettelheim can be found below

http://www.hagalil.com/2010/03/bettelheim-spiegel/

However, the author sees behind the attacks rather anti-Semitic attitude, which I can not share so.

4   Mixing science and parenthood

Until the "fridge mother" myth, which, according to the hypothesis, was intentionally and maliciously set against all facts, science and parenting were separate. And scientists were experts because of their training and applied critical methods.

The myth discredited not only Bettelheim, but the whole science!

„For many in the autism community, the popularity of the refrigerator-mother hypothesis before the 1970s continues to be remembered as an example of what might be called "the tyranny of expertise"—the danger of giving professionals too much power." [Baker (2010)]

Parenting and science were mixed, with parents claiming and taking the expertise to this day. And that without factual basis.

Through the lobbying and financing of studies, the parent associations were suddenly the principals and masters in the House of Science. There was no resistance from the scientists who readily left the soil of science. And that with devastating consequences for autistic people, but also their parents [see also: Schmidt (2015)].

4.1   Narcissism

The best thing about Rimland's theory in connection with the ASA is that it satisfies the narcissism of the parents.

„Rimland postulates that "Children stricken with early infantile autismas a primary disorder were genetically

vulnerable to autism as a consequence of an inborn capacity for high intelligence." This statement is based on Kanner's original observations on the intelligence of the parents of autistic children. ...

The parents of the thirty-nine remaining cases distribute themselves as follows: In eleven cases, one or both parents may be considered of better-than-average, and possibly of superior intelligence. Only one parent, a father, showed intelligence and achievement that we would generally acknowledge to be superior, since he is a scientist of international reputation. None of the others have shown achievements that would lift them out of the ordinary. There are two physicians among them, two lawyers, and one college teacher; thus the intellectual professions are well represented in this group. For the twenty-eight remaining children the story is different, all their parents being of average intelligence. ...

This leaves a parental ratio of thirty-four average to eleven sets of better than average or superior intelligence, only one of whom has shown outstanding achievement-hardly an impressive validation of the alleged superior intelligence of parents of autistic children. Among our group of thirty-four sets of parents of average or below-average intelligence are day laborers (two of them more often than not unemployed), farmhands, a post-office clerk, but also one high school

58

teacher, two accountants, etc. The largest single category is of people in business who are either self-employed or salaried (seven parents), followed by white-collar workers (four)." [Bettelheim (1967)]

And Rimland at the same time takes all the parents' responsibility - to immediately put them back on the parents' shoulders via ABA. "If you do not ABA with your child, you deny him his chances!" So to speak or similar is the credo of the autism parent associations.

But even with respect to the supposedly high intelligence in the parents of autistics, Bettelheim turns out to be a tough critic:

„Until such time as a large random sample of the population will have been studied as to the incidence of infantile autism, it is my opinion that we ought to disregard claims as to the ethnic origin of such children, and as to their parents' superior intelligence and professional achievements. This is because the sample that comes to the attention of child psychiatrists is much too skewed by factors I have mentioned (which parents keep autistic chiklren alive, which of them are not satisfied with the still common diagnosis of feeble-mindedness and/or brain damage, which ones seek

psychiatric evaluation for their children, and so on)."
[Bettelheim (1967)]

5   Distortion of the facts

The misrepresentations regarding Bettelheim and the
"fridge mother" are still pervading the media and also the
"science". Et al on en.wikipedia.org there is a wrong
representation:

*„Rimland published his book, Infantile Autism: The
Syndrome and Its Implications for a Neural Theory of
Behavior, in 1964. Its foreword, by Leo Kanner, the man
who first identified autism as a syndrome, gave the book
credibility among professionals in the field. It was an
about-turn for Kanner, the originator of the word
"autism" and of the "refrigerator mother" theory;
through his observations and research, Kanner had come
to believe that autism had a neurological cause—the
accepted view in the medical profession today. But at the
time Rimland's book was published, and for many years
afterwards, a common theory was that autism was
caused by unloving 'refrigerator mothers', an unproven
but widely accepted idea most famously propounded by
University of Chicago professor Bruno Bettelheim,
notably in his book The Empty Fortress: Infantile Autism*

and the Birth of the Self (1967), which claimed that the traumatized unloved child retreated into autism. As a professional research psychologist, Rimland was well positioned to launch the first major attack on Bettelheim's theory. Rimland's was the first authoritative voice to dispute Bettelheim's research and call into question his conclusions.

Parents from all over the United States, excited that, for the first time, a professional in the field did not accuse them of maltreating their autistic child, began to write to Rimland. He called a meeting in Teaneck, New Jersey, at the house of one of the families, and this small group of parents, including Ruth C. Sullivan (first president of the ASA), became the nucleus that founded the Autism Society of America." [Quelle: en.wikipedia.org]

But only the time sequence questions the presentation: Rimland's book "Infantile Autism" was published in 1964.
The ASA was u.a. founded by Rimland and Lovaas in 1965.
Bettelheim's "Empty Fortress" appeared in 1967 with clear criticism of both Rimland's position and ABA.
The Autism Research Institute was also founded by Rimland in 1967.

Not only that in "The Empty Fortress", which is always mentioned as a source, is more evidence against the "fridge mother" myth than for it, the order is not correct! And Bettelheim explicitly states that he is right about Rimland in the point that it is not good to blame the parents!

VI. LOOK BACK

From today's perspective, Bettelheim was on the right path. If this path had been pursued further in research, it probably would not have taken until 2015 before a first comprehensive, socio-psychological / development-dynamic theory was developed.
A primitive biologic approach, beyond scientific methodology, has prevailed.

"The impact of the book was dramatic. In 1978, a national magazine reported that 90 percent of the people in the field felt that Rimland had 'blown Bettelheim's theories to hell.' I have often been told that Infantile Autism was pivotal in redirecting the entire field of psychology from its morbid preoccupation with psychodynamics toward a more productive interest in biology. While my two main goals, exposing the psycho-genie myth and encouraging biological research, were realized, my attempt to clarify the muddled problem of diagnosing autism has had little success."
[aus: This Week's Citation Classic, CC/NUMBER 22, JUNE 1, 1981]

At that time a differentiated scientific activity and a massive defamation faced each other.
As is known and not surprising, the defamation has won.
A resistance on the part of science is unknown to me.
The consequences to date have been over 50 years of standstill in the understanding of autism and in the support of autistics.
And science has not only lost its independence, but also its innocence.

„Verliert eine Wissenschaft nicht an Glaubwürdigkeit, wenn sie vermeidet, auch ihren Ansichten wider- sprechende Erfahrungen zu diskutieren?"
[Stork, Jochen, Vorwort zu Bettelheim (1967)
„Does not a science lose credibility if it avoids discussing its conflicting experiences?"]

It simply turned the relationship between science and ignorance upside down.

*„In 1964, the release of Dr. Bernard Rimland's book, Infantile Autism, revolutionized the autism field by providing the autism community with much-needed guidance on how to understand and treat individuals on the spectrum. He single-handedly realigned the field from a psychodynamic, **parent-blaming** perspective to a*

64

scientific, physiological course of action. This 50th anniversary edition presents the original book with contributions from leaders in the autism field, including Drs. Martha Herbert and Simon Baron-Cohen, who celebrate Dr. Rimland's exceptional work, and place his findings within the context of autism as we understand it today. Bringing Dr. Rimland's findings up to date for a new generation of readers, this book will be fascinating reading for parents and those on the autism spectrum as well as professionals working with autism and anyone with an interest in autism and/or psychological theory."
[Blurb to the issue of the 50th anniversary of Rimland (1964)]

No, the psychodynamic approach was and is not "parent-blaming"!
And no, the exclusive physiological approach alone has nothing to do with science.
And no, parents do not have any comparable expertise with scientists!

1   Science turns into a dangerous myth

"Myth turns into dangerous error when it stops the search for knowledge by lulling us into thinking a problem is solved when in fact it is not even recognized.

65

The problem I refer to, of course, is that of infantile autism. There are many ways in which it goes unrecognized, one of the oldest being to consider these children feeble-minded or brain-damaged. But even this belief is very young compared to the ancient one that they were mothered by animals." [Bettelheim (1967)]

The myth of the "fridge mother" and the discrediting of science and the scientist Bettelheim led to 50 years of standstill in autism research. In addition, generations of parents have taken the hope for a positive development of their autistic children.

*„Among the purposes of this book is to do away with a few widely held notions about autistic children which we believe to be in error. Because in science especially, the correction of error can often do more to solve a thorny problem than some new discovery or theory. **Often, too, erroneous ideas can keep the valid knowledge we already have from being put into use.** The knowledge I refer to is what we already know about autistic children. **In preceding chapters I have presented the bases for our conviction that these children are not feeble-minded, but suffer from a disturbance we believe to be functional and which we know to be reversible in many***

cases, if treated early and radically enough."
[Bettelheim (1967)]

Today we can say with certainty that Bettelheim was
right with this statement!

1.1   Restriction of Therapeutic Approaches

Bettelheim's aim, and it should have been made clear,
was not to accuse parents or blaming them for anything.
Bettelheim wanted to find ways to help autistic children.

*„Wherever infantile autism is viewed as an inborn
impairment, of whatever variety, the resultant attitudes
toward treatment will be defeatist. Among those, on the
other hand, who trace the causes of autism at least in
part to the environmental influence, outlooks will be
more optimistic because of the not always valid but
convincing belief that what environment has caused,
environment may also be able to correct.
Nor is the pessimism limited to those who embrace the
organic hypothesis. Study of the literature suggests it is
also dominant among many who accept a psychogenic
hypothesis, even in part. In my opinion the pessimism is
unwarranted and may be ascribed to the fact that all too
few efforts at treatment were intensive enough, and even*

more important, were sustained for the requisite number of years. Thus when Kanner [1954a] and Kanner and Lesser [1958], state that infantile autism has not been influenced by any form of therapy, I can only explain it by the fact that the therapy was not appropriate in terms of methods used, or of intensiveness or duration of treatment. " [Bettelheim (1967)]

And he stands in clear contrast to Rimland, which excludes treatment options beyond ABA from the outset.

„Rimland shares none of Kanner's doubts, but states apodictically that "no form of psychiatric treatment has been known to alter the course of aurism." How right or wrong he is the reader will have to decide after reading the case histories in this volume, or if he goes to the trouble of reading some of the sources Rimland refers to himself. For example, he quotes Eveloff [1960] five times in support of his own theories, but fails to mention that Eveloff's is a report on the excellent progress of a three-and-a-half-year-old autistic girl after only several months of outpatient treatment. (Though the therapist favored placement in a treatment institution, he was opposed in this suggestion by the parents.) Nor does Rimland mention that Eveloff concludes his article by saying: "There is no question that she has improved

greatly, and there is considerable evidence to support the contention that this improvement is the result of psychiatric treatment."
Rimland asserts further that "recovery in those cases where it has occurred, has apparently been spontaneous" and that chances for such recovery are slight. Whether, for example, Marcia's recovery, or Joey s, were spontaneous or the result of intensive treatment the reader will have his own chance to decide. "
[Bettelheim (1967)]

Was it the goal or consequence of discrediting Bettelheim, only ABA remained as a treatment option. A rogue who thinks badly at the connection of Rimland and Lovaas (as the "father" of ABA).

1.2   ABA as supposed "gold standard"

Until today, completely wrongly and because of massive propaganda of the parent organizations like ASA and "Autism Speaks", but also "Autismus Deutschland", ABA is considered the "gold standard" in the treatment of early childhood autism. There was no significant development in this area in 50 years.
The supposed "evidence base" is pseudoscientific humbug, as already stated in Schmidt (2016).

For the sake of completeness we have to mention TECCH and PECS, but they also lack the understanding of what autism is and that autistics are not on a par with animals.

Alternatives such as child-centered approaches, which we have presented in Ganz, A .; Schmidt, B. J. (2016) and are very similar to the basic idea of Bettelheim, have so far simply been unjustly ignored.

VII.   OUTLOOK

It is imperative that scientific principles in autism
research be reintroduced.
This includes the discussion of conflicting theories. The
permanent "Semmelweis reflex" [see: Schmidt (2016)]
should be eliminated.

Also regarding possible support programs for autistic
people, child-centered approaches need to be given
critical attention and readiness to develop.
Further, a social change is necessary, for, as Vygotsky
(1929) correctly writes:

*„Thus, the task is not so much the education of blind
children as it is the reeducation of the sighted. The latter
must change their attitude toward blindness and toward
the blind. The reeducation of the sighted poses a social
pedagogical task of enormous importance."*

And that's the same with autism!

Parents and self-help groups are important, but have far
less than their claimed expertise.

BIBLIOGRAPHY

Baker, Jeffrey P. (2010): Autism in 1959: Joey the mechanical boy. In: Pediatrics 125 (6), S. 1101–1103. DOI: 10.1542/peds.2010-0846.

Bettelheim, Bruno (1967): The Empty Fortress: Infantile Autism and the Birth of the Self.

Bettelheim, Bruno (1950): Love is Not Enough-the Treatment of Emotionally Disturbed Children. 1. edition. the free press, glencoe, illinois

Bettelheim Bruno (1985): Erziehung zum Überleben. Zur Psychologie der Extremsituation. 2. Auflage. Stuttgart: Deutsche Verlags-Anstalt.

Frith, Uta (1989): Explaining the enigma.

Ganz, Andreas; Schmidt, Bernhard J. (2016): Klartext kompakt. Frühkindlicher Autismus: Verstehen = Helfen. Norderstedt: Books on Demand (Klartext kompakt, 8).

Khoziev, Vadim B.; Schmidt, Bernhard J. (2017): Auf der Suche nach einer Autismus-Theorie. Ein Russisch-Deutscher Dialog. 1. Auflage. Norderstedt: Books on Demand.

Rimland, Bernard (1964): Infantile Autism. The syndrome and its implications for a neural theory of behavior

Schmidt, Bernhard J. (2015):
Autistic and Society - An angry change of perspective: Volume 1: Understanding Autism
Norderstedt: Books on Demand.

Schmidt, Bernhard J. (2016):
Autismus. Wenn Händewaschen hilft. Norderstedt: Books on Demand.

Schmidt, Bernhard J.; Ganz, Andreas (2016):
Plaintext compact. The Asperger Syndrome: Not only for Psychotherapists. Norderstedt: Books on Demand.

Vygotskij, Lev Semenovič (1929); in Rieber, Robert W.; Carton, Aaron S. (op. 1987-): The collected works of L.S. Vygotsky. New York: Plenum Press (Cognition and language).

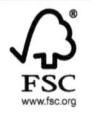